DEDICATION

This book is dedicated to Eric. My home is your home. You are always welcome to come back after you have travelled the world.

TABLE OF CONTENTS

Healthy Eating Training for the Young

Weight Loss and Management Basics for Kids

By: Nancy Green

9781635014907

PUBLISHERS NOTES

Disclaimer – Speedy Publishing LLC

This publication is intended to provide helpful and informative material. It is not intended to diagnose, treat, cure, or prevent any health problem or condition, nor is intended to replace the advice of a physician. No action should be taken solely on the contents of this book. Always consult your physician or qualified health-care professional on any matters regarding your health and before adopting any suggestions in this book or drawing inferences from it.

The author and publisher specifically disclaim all responsibility for any liability, loss or risk, personal or otherwise, which is incurred as a consequence, directly or indirectly, from the use or application of any contents of this book.

Any and all product names referenced within this book are the trademarks of their respective owners. None of these owners have sponsored, authorized, endorsed, or approved this book.

Always read all information provided by the manufacturers' product labels before using their products. The author and publisher are not responsible for claims made by manufacturers.

This book was originally printed before 2014. This is an adapted reprint by Speedy Publishing LLC with newly updated content designed to help readers with much more accurate and timely information and data.

Speedy Publishing LLC

40 E Main Street, Newark, Delaware, 19711

Contact Us: 1-888-248-4521

Website: http://www.speedypublishing.co

REPRINTED Paperback Edition: 9781635014907:

Manufactured in the United States of America

Chapter 1- A Healthy Diet for a Healthy Child

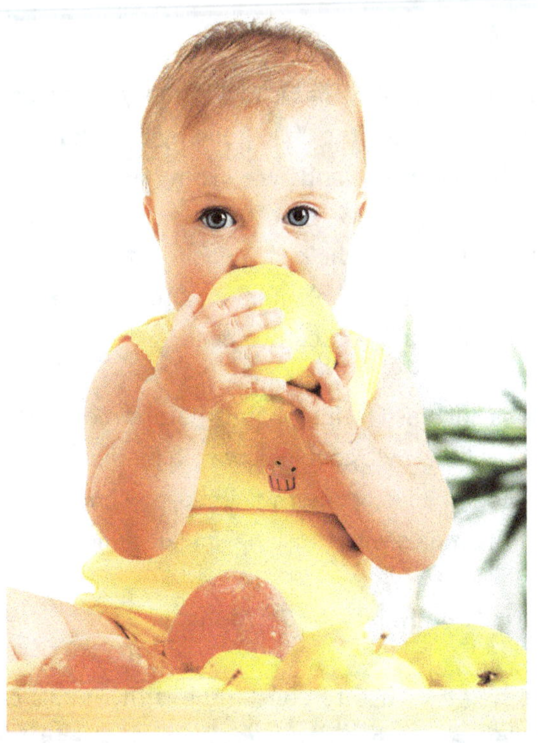

Generally a healthy child is one that is less likely to be susceptible to any diseases or sicknesses that may be going around at the time. Most children are able to live a happy and healthy life with the help of a good diet plan and the daily physical activity that will help them function optimally both mentally and physically.

Keeping the child healthy is really the responsibility of the parent as is teaching the child to adopt good habit that will help keep the child from being unnecessarily exposed to anything unhealthy.

However should there be a need to address any less than desirable health conditions, it may be prudent to seek medical advice at the earliest possible stage.

There are also possibilities of using a more holistic approach to treating mild infections as it is not always good to pump a child with pills and medicine that may have long term residual side effects.

Besides a healthy diet plan that is nutritionally balanced, the parent would also need to teach the child good hygiene habits. This should be practiced both at home and away from home.

Good hygiene will also help to ensure the child is not left susceptible to negative elements through habit that may encourage such prevailing circumstances.

Simple actions such as washing hands before meals and also when using public facilities, will go a long way in helping to keep the child safe from being exposed to germs. Children should also be taught to avoid sharing meals with those having any kind of infections.

Forming Good Food Habits While Young

However getting the child to consume healthy meals can often be quite a challenge and healthy means usually mean uninteresting and bland food to the child mostly distorted taste buds.

Children usually enjoyed foods that are very flavorful, sweet or simply not really healthy for them. However with some research and proper planning it is possible to design a complete diet plan that is nutritionally balanced to suit various age groups the children may fall into.

Getting the full range of proteins, iron, calcium and vitamin A should ideally be the focus of the diet plan in place. When it comes to the appetite of children, there will usually be noticeable fluctuations and this will be reflected according to the growth the child is experiencing at any particular juncture in their lives.

Ideally a general gauge to go by would be that most 3 year olds would need about 1300 calories daily, while a 10 year old would need about 2000 calories daily and the adolescent would need 2800 calories a day.

Including a healthy amount of vegetables, fruits, dairy products, meats and beans would be ideal when it comes to trying to provide for a complete dietary plan. Snacks are also fine but should be nutritionally based too.

The Food Pyramid

Most children require the same basic nutritional needs that are going to help with their bodies needs for optimal growth. Therefore it would be wise for the parents to explore the merits of understanding and providing healthy food options based on the ideal food pyramid for children.

Basically the food pyramid will consists of five ideal yet very different food categories and these would include fruits, vegetable, grains, oils and meats and beans.

By taking the time and effort to understand the nutrients in each of the different food groups, the parent will be able to determine how much is needed from each type for the child's daily consumption needs.

This will also help the parent come up with a complete and effective nutritional diet plan for the child to follow. This will also help to decrease the chances of the child becoming obese which seems to be the current trend today among children all over the world.

The food pyramid should ideally start with the bottom being the main source of overall energy food that should be items such as corn, potatoes, healthy breads, pasta, rice, and legumes.

The next level up should come in two separate categories where group one would ideally consists of all kinds of vegetables while group two would be based on various different fresh fruits.

The third level of the pyramid would also have to be divided into two categories where one would represent of the dairy based products while the other would consists of various meats, fish and eggs. The last level at the top of the pyramid should consist of controlled amounts of fats, oil, sugar and salt. This last category should be carefully monitored as it is not really altogether very healthy but nonetheless necessary.

Reducing Sugar and Flour Intake

Basically not known for its healthy qualities, being able to eliminate large portions of flour and sugar from a child's basic diet plan would be an ideal goal to work towards. These ingredients do little to promote healthy and wholesome growth in children of any ages, thus consciously eliminating these from the diet plan would be a step in the right direction.

It would be a good and sensible idea to adopt a lesser intake if these two items from the very start, as the idea of flour and sugar in the child daily intake would not really benefit in any way except perhaps to enhance flavor and volume in the foods eaten.

Nancy Green
This elimination or control will help the child achieve a more healthy weight gain percentage and overall healthier body condition.

Optimal weight conditions usually means the connecting optimal number of calorie intake and with the reduction of flour and sugar in the diet plan this ideal platform can be easily achieved.

Ideally the high calorie items such as breads should be replaced with low calorie items such as legumes that will also help to keep the child satisfied for longer periods of time.

Other alternative would be replacing sugar with the more healthy option of honey as this too will help to cut down on the unnecessary high calorie intake.

Eating food items such as oatmeal, fresh fruits, grains and nuts would certainly be better than breads, jams, pancakes and other sweetened foods that may be satisfying but for only a short time.

Avoiding high intakes of sugar and flour in the daily diet plan of a child will also help the child to have a healthier future as an adult. Good habit formed as a child will usually follow on through adulthood, thus eating healthy from the start would be an ideal plan to go with.

The Dangers of Fats to the Young

Generally it is an accepted fact that every child needs some amount of fats within the daily diet plan as these fats contribute to the energy levels that gives the body what it needs to work in a healthy manner. However too much of the fat intake will eventually effect the body system in ways that are eventually damaging to the child's eventual growth and health.

Healthy Eating Training for the Young
Children who make it a habit of consuming high fat diets will eventually cause the unhealthy fats like saturated fats and trans fats to clog the arteries, thus adding to the disruptive blood flow for the body's needs.

This will then lead to the higher possibility of sustaining heart problems as the child grows older. Current statistics show that more people are having some form of heart problems at much earlier stages in the life.

There is also some significant connection between the fats intake and the presence of cancer cell in the body system. Saturated fats have been the significant cause for concern as it is touted to be the main cause of cancer cells multiplying at faster rates within the body.

Obesity is also another unhealthy side effect caused by the large amounts of uncontrolled fat intake for children.

Children are usually seeking out foods that will give them immediate satisfaction and these usually take on the unhealthy features of junk food or other snacks that are not based on healthy nutritional values.

This obese condition will then lead to other medical complications such as gallbladder disease, fatty liver disease, gastro esophageal reflux, sleep apnea, gout and osteoarthritis as the child grows into adulthood.

There is also the added risk of sustaining type 2 diabetes even as a child, especially if the child is not active in sports and outdoor activities.

Nancy Green
Don't Take Out the Fun in Eating

Most parent lament of the problems they have to deal with when it comes of children who are generally fussy eaters. However it is possible to be able to get child to consume healthy foods if they are presented in a fun manner and are delicious tasting. Therefore it would really be up to the parent to make the effort to find innovative and interesting ways to ensure the child willing eats healthy foods or snacks.

Most children diligently avoid the food group that is centered on vegetable, thus creating huge problems for parents who are well aware of the merits of this food group and how much it will benefit their child.

Making a simple carrot stick more appealing to the child would require some effort on the part of the parent which may take the form of making the consumption of such a food group an activity that is part of a game or even cutting the carrot to resemble fun items such as animal shapes.

Getting the child to participate in the preparation process of preparing the meal or snack will help the child feel a sense of achievement, and this will encourage the child to also want to try the foods prepared by themselves or at least where they have actually participated in the preparation.

This sense of achievement can be a good and effective tool to use to get the child to eat healthy as the fun ingredient can be a very persuasive encouragement.

Children tend to eat with the eyes first and then their tongues, meaning that if the food does not look appealing, getting them to even taste it would be an uphill battle. Therefore including a lot of color into the presentation would be one way of creating an appealing palate for the child.

Chapter 2- The Dangers of Obesity

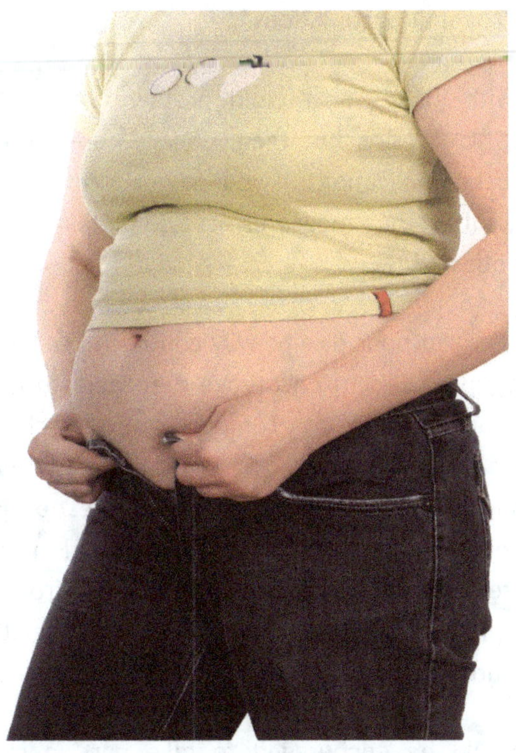

Obesity in teenagers and children is maybe one of the saddest sights I see. It is cruel and horrible for children to be that overweight, and they will not have a good social life or medical life, and many things will get them down. They will find it hard to make friends as they will be bullied at school due to their weight and their health will suffer greatly as medical complications are always paired with obesity. We need to help our children and out teenagers to shake their unhealthy lives and get back into fitness and healthy living!

Factors that Contribute to Obesity

Teen obesity is a great complicated problem, as obesity is not always caused by laziness and over eating; it is sometimes due to their family's medical history and medical conditions that they may be suffering. Although not all teen obesity is due to genetics, it can also be due to medical conditions.

Problems with glands or thyroid problems are often a cause contributing to obesity, but then, obesity contributes too many other medical complications. If you do not want to see your child or teenager suffer, then measures need to be taken to sort out the problem of obesity!

Albeit laziness and poor diet heavily contribute to the problem of teen obesity, we need to encourage teenagers to get out more, instead of playing inside with computers and watching television. They need to be shown what an acceptable diet is, and taught that junk food and convenience foods are not the best option for them, and that there are healthy alternatives available! In doing this you help fight teen obesity and save our children from a future of emotional problems, and most importantly health problems associated with obesity.

Children should be encouraged to take part in more physical activities such as sports and going out more. This will ensure the burning of more calories than they are eating; therefore keeping the weight off and, if needed, they will lose the weight they need to lose.

Parents need to take a stand to help prevent teen obesity and get their children "sorted out." For all that they say that you can take a horse to water but you can't make it drink, healthy eating should be demonstrated by the parents and the children will follow their lead! Teenagers should be made aware of the consequences of obesity and helped towards a better future!

Nancy Green
Genetics May Play a Part

In some instances, some people claim that genetics can play a major part in childhood obesity. It does, but not as big as the role that parents' mindset and influence do. It is a falsehood that genetic materials induce a child to be heavy at an early age.

For the greater part of the population, genetic materials may establish the lower maximum values of people's weight, but people themselves establish the higher maximum values, by their food choices. In addition, since most kids cannot simply set the limits and choose the food that they need to eat, it is the duty of the parents to set the limits.

Chapter 3- The Obese Child

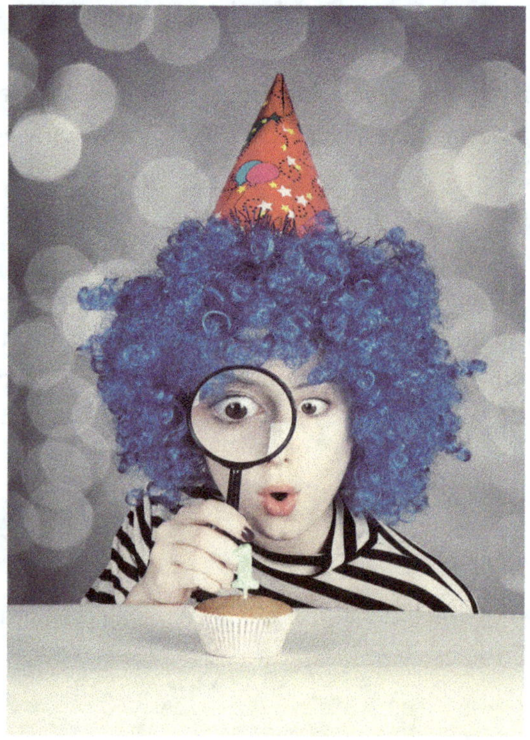

Obesity is supposed to be categorized as the unhealthy overweight condition in the human body and when this becomes apparent at a very young age such as in children, the parents should take a serious look at the diet plan and daily lifestyle of the child as these are probably the two main factors contributing to this negative condition.

The calorie intake should ideally be matched with the amount being burnt off during physical activity and when the intake is more than the required amount the effective burning of these excess becomes harder to manage thus allowing accumulation to set in.

This of course then brings the individual to the point of becoming obese. Ideally the child's lifestyle should center on the ability to burn off more calories than the actual intake.

The following are some ways parent can adopt when trying to keep the likelihood of their child becoming obese in check:

At the stage of infancy, breastfeeding would be an ideal option to choose and delaying the introduction of solid food into the daily dietary plan for the child would be advised. Studies have shown that this delay would help in preventing obesity from occurring early on in the child's life.

Children should be encouraged to only consume healthy foods, and this should extend to all types of categories such as snacks, main meals and any other form of food consumption. Making it a habit to serve only low fat snacks while also encouraging the child to be active and adopt some form of daily physical activity would ideally keep the child from becoming obese.

Begin Burning Fats with a Good Breakfast

The importance of breakfast should never be taken for granted as the energy that provides for optimal mental and physical health starts with a good healthy breakfast plan.

Breakfast is a good way to get the body's system awake and off to a good working start as it help to refuel the body after the long rest.

It has been noted that children who eat breakfast tend to eat healthier overall and are more likely to participate in physical activities and are mentally alert, thus allowing the child the opportunity for healthy growth.

Skipping breakfast can usually cause the child to be irritable, tired, restless and basically distracted and unable to get both their body and mind in sync to get through the day effectively and productively. The mood and energy levels will usually drop by mid-morning if there is no proper breakfast intake daily.

Being one of the ideal ways to kick start the mind and body, breakfast also contributes to the healthy body metabolism rate that allows the body to process and convert the foods into fuel for the energy required for optimal function throughout the day.

When the metabolism rate get moving, the body will then be able to start burning the calories effectively thus decreasing the likelihood of fat build ups within the body system.

It has been noted that children who are not consistent with the regiment of nutritional breakfast intake generally frequently snack on unhealthy foods during the day, thus causing them to become overweight easily.

Choosing breakfast food that are rich in whole grains, fiber and protein while at the same time low in added sugar will help to boost the child's attention span, concentration and memory retention processes, all of which are crucial element for being able to focus and absorb what is being taught in school.

Oatmeal Helps Reduce Weight

Did you know that simply eating breakfast raises your metabolism by 10 percent?

Oatmeal is one of the most powerful breakfast foods of them all. If you are looking to get your body in great shape, you should incorporate this as a staple food in your diet. Oatmeal is the perfect meal to start your day because it boosts your energy and has plenty of fiber to keep you full and satisfied. Oatmeal breaks down slowly in the stomach, giving you long-lasting energy. It is also full of water soluble fibers, which play a crucial role in making you feel full over a longer period of time.

Studies have also shown that oatmeal reduces cholesterol, maintains blood sugar levels and fights against heart disease, diabetes, colon cancer, and obesity.

If you want to add some powerful antioxidants to your oatmeal, simply throw on some blueberries and raspberries. These delicious fruits are packed with antioxidants that fight against heart disease, cancer, and a multitude of other ailments. Blueberries have also been proven to preserve vision. This powerful fruit rated highest in antioxidants among over 40 fruits and vegetables.

However, oatmeal doesn't just have to be for breakfast. You can use it a couple hours before you exercise to energize your workout. You can even include oatmeal in your smoothies. It is also a wonderful addition to muffins and even as a covering for chicken breasts. Keep in mind that you must buy the unsweetened, unflavored variety.

To spice it up a little, you can use bananas, berries, or milk. The downfall of pre-flavored oatmeal is that it often comes loaded with sugar calories. So, stick to the good stuff. You will get all the beneficial energy for your sports and activities, and none of the bad effects of sugar.

If you're looking for oatmeal with a little more texture, you can try out the steel-cut oat variety. Although this type does take a little longer to cook, I find that it is well worth the wait. They have a somewhat chewier texture and heartier flavor than rolled oats. Once you try this variety, you may never go back.

If you're having trouble with late night binges, have a bowl of oatmeal instead. This will help squash your cravings. Not to mention, you'll be avoiding any junk food or empty calories. If you're looking to get in the best shape of your life, I suggest your alternate your morning meals between oatmeal on one day and have eggs and meat on another. This will put your fat-burning into overdrive.

Studies: Obesity Leads to Injuries

So, if you are in the teen ages and feel troubled by those extra inches around your waist, don't wait any further to embrace a suitable weight loss programs for teens that you think works well for your body.

Get your act together today! Given below are few invaluable teen weight loss tips, as seen in many of the best weight loss programs for teens, prescribed by expert nutritionists, which could help you to take on the fight with your foe – overweight.

Therefore, the best weight loss programs for teens must include a suggestion to the teen, to control the daily intake of food, especially fatty and oily foodstuff. Also take care to avoid milk products, all sorts of junk foods, and artificial drinks.

Another aspect that best weight loss programs for teens suggest is to drink lots of water and incorporate fruits, raw vegetables, and fibrous foods into the diet. It is vital in balancing the nutrient content in the body caused due to the reduction in the normal intake (assuming you are following the first suggestion, as such).

Nancy Green

Replace your normal snacks – such as a packet of chips or potato wafers – with something that is healthier to your system. That is, substitute your chips or other fat and oil rich snacks with something like:

• Frozen grapes

• Cherry tomatoes

• Baby carrots

• Low-fat pudding or yogurt

But, the most important of all the suggestions is that you must nurture a strong will to follow the diet program you choose, religiously. Else, no best weight loss programs for teens could help you bring down your weight.

Chapter 4- The Importance of Physical Activity

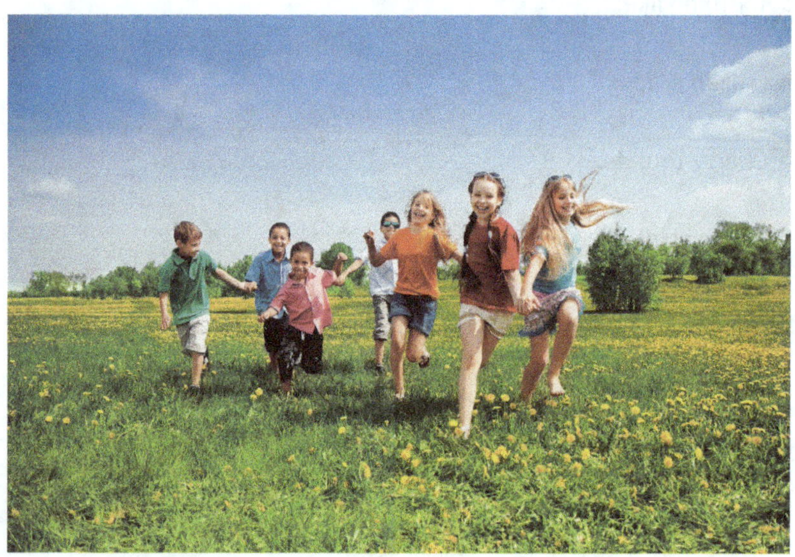

Take a few hours every day to work out in the gym or spend some time running or playing your favorite sport. Such physical activities could burn away those extra calories from under your skin! In fact, this is the most important step one could find in all the best weight loss programs for teens, suggested by experts.

Having an active child is almost always a good sign as this would signify that the child is well adjusted and happy. It would also mean that the child is growing well and hopefully able to access to a well-balanced and nutritional diet plan. Rest and proper exercise will help the child to grow into a healthy, happy and mentally alert child.

Children should be encouraged to have a lot of physical activity in the daily life as this will contribute positively to the stronger muscles and bone conditions.

It will also ensure the child is less likely to be become overweight. The risk of contracting a number of diseases will also be significantly decreased when the body condition is healthy due to the adequate amount of exercise it is conditioned to experience.

Exercising regularly as a child will also help the child to have this same positive habit through into the adult phase in life too, thus giving the body the opportunity to be fit and healthy always.

Taking the importance of exercise for granted and not incorporating a suitable regiment into the lifestyle of the child will eventually cause the child to experience alto of medical complications that will severely interrupt the child's ability to lead a healthy life.

An hour a day would be an ideal target time frame for vigorous physical activity. This could be in the form of sports, games, jogging in the park or simply brisk walking to and from school.

Rest is also another important element that should be part of the child's daily regimen of the healthy lifestyle.

Having an active exercise routine will help the child sleep better and thus contribute toward better overall body and mind conditions. An adequate amount of sleep will allow the child to be better prepared to face the day and both body and mind would have enjoyed adequate rest.

Limit TV and Gadgets Time

Trying to limit the access a child has to TV and the internet can be a challenge especially if this course of action is rather sudden. Therefore is would be advisable for the parent to start the limitations from a very early age and use other more beneficial activities as a possible positive distraction.

Given the opportunity most children today would rather opt to watch their favorite TV program or surf the internet indefinitely as such prolonged viewing are certainly made possible on both platforms.

The following are some ways that can be effectively used to lure the child's attention away from these rarely beneficial activities to something more productive mentally and physically:

Placing the TV or internet access in an area where there is a lot of activity will help to keep distraction levels high thus making it quite difficult to indulge in either of these activities for long.

Also ensuring there are a lot of other activities and entertainment possibilities such as board games and books so that the child will have options available to explore instead of just the TV or internet.

Setting a daily allowance for watching TV or surfing the internet would also be something to consider. Once this daily quota is exhausted, the child should be strictly encouraged to seek other forms of entertainment preferably something that involved some kind of outdoor activity.

To ensure this is made more interesting, parent participation would be encouraged as this will make the child feel wanted and thus make the whole exercise more enjoyable.

Making TV or internet access something that should be earned rather than something that is there for the taking is another effective method of limiting access to both.

Nancy Green

Allowing the child access to either of these, only after chores and homework has been completed will not only encourage responsibility and discipline but will also help the child understand the merits of rewards.

CHAPTER 5- KEEP HEALTH INSURANCE

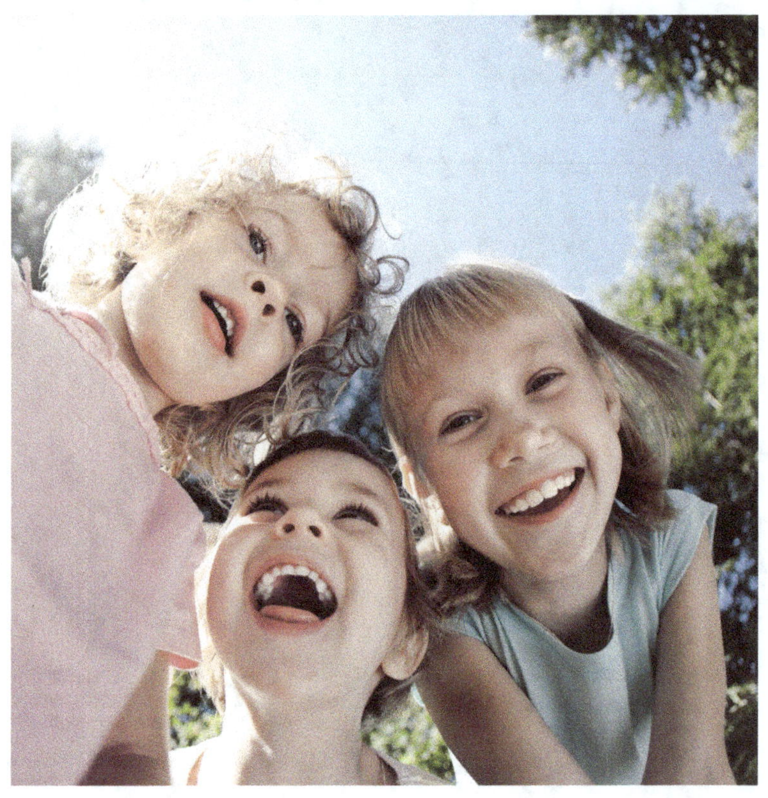

Insurance for children is very rarely contemplated as an important facility to have on hand. This is mainly due to the fact that most insurance companies don't really push or promote these kinds of packages to their clients. However as the cost of medical fees escalate; it would be something that the parent should be prepared to seriously consider should the need to medical attention become necessary.

There are probably several different programs and policies available in the market today and the parent would ideally have to take the opportunity to explore as many options as possible before making an informed decision.

There is also the long term cost incurred for any insurance policy taken up, as most policies will be considered null or inactive if the payments defaults.

Therefore understanding, that this is effectively a rather long commitment for the parent is crucial to deciding which policy is most suited for the child and the household budget.

The method of making claims on the insurance policy for the child is also important. The parent should read and understand all clauses hidden and otherwise before choosing to sign on to a particular policy being advertised.

There would also be a need for the parent to enquire at the local hospital the acceptance outline in place should the child need medical assistance immediately by with the use of the insurance.

Ensuring the hospital is willing and able to accept the insurance coverage to facilitate the medical procedures needed should be established before committing to the policy.

In spite of all the various elements that should be checked and rechecked before actually committing to a particular policy for the health of the child, it is still better to have a medical health insurance policy, as this will definitely ensure the parent is able to consider more costly medical options should there be a need to do so.

Although there are several different diseases a child will commonly be exposed to, these can be prevented with the adequate amount of good hygiene practices firmly in place. But in spite of all the possible precautions taken, the child may still fall prey to these diseases so knowledge is extremely important.

The following are some of the more common childhood disease:

Respiratory syncytial virus – being a rather common disease which is further enhanced with the presence of the flu bug, it usually causes a lot of problems for the child.

These would include pneumonia and bronchiolitis, inflammation of the small air passages in the lungs, and general difficulty in breathing.

Fifth disease or otherwise known as slapped cheek disease – this is usually seen as a lacy red rash that would appear on the child's torso and limbs.

Although the child may not experience and severe life threatening possibilities, nonetheless it is a rather uncomfortable experience especially for younger children.

Hand, foot and mouth disease – this is considered a rather common disease where blisters or sores will appear inside the mouth and on the palms of the hands and also on the soles of the feet.

The virus that causes this disease will create a lot of discomfort for the child but is not really serious and will usually decapitate after about 10 days.

Scarlet fever or otherwise sometimes also known as strep throat – this infection is usually cause the child to experience severe soreness in the throat area accompanied by a bout of high fever.

The scarlet fever rash usually starts on the chest and then extends to the abdomen and then all over the body. It usually has the look similar to that of bright red sunburn patches.

How to Boost Your Child's Immunity

Healthy and happy children are less likely to succumb easily to diseases as their immune system would be strong enough to be able to withstand and onslaught of negativity.

Any child will be able to function better if he or she has been taught to adhere to clean and tidy attitudes and environments. Encouraging the child to have a regular exercise program or physical activity will also help to further strengthen to possibility of having the long term enjoyment that good health conditions can bring.

With the proper foundation in place the child will also be able to avoid any instances of obesity and ill health which seems to be quite common today. This is mostly due to the very unhealthy diet plans and lifestyle most children indulge in.

Parents should take the practice of preparing healthy meals so that the children can develop this habit and carry it on into adulthood.

Exercising with the child will also help the child understand the merits of this with regard to maintaining long term good health.

Doing these things together will also have the added benefit of creating a closer bond between parent and child, thus effectively allowing the child to feel loved and wanted always.

CHAPTER 6- HOW TO HELP YOU CHILD FIGHT OBESITY

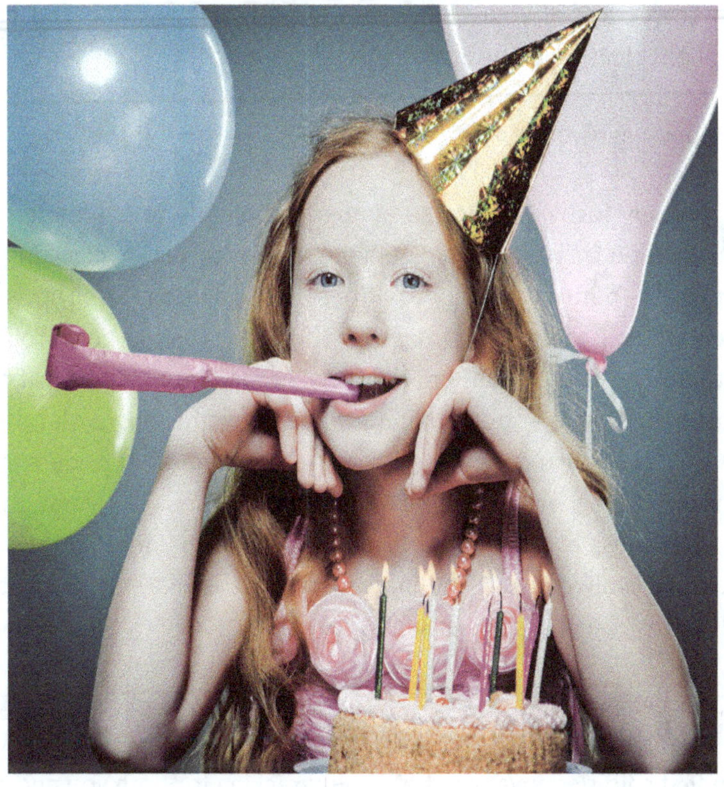

Halloween, slumber parties, birthdays —sometimes, it seems like childhood is one humongous food fest!

It is difficult to deprive your child with special delicacies and delights when all her friends are having a grand feast. However, this simple condition can bring about more trouble than you can think of. Treating your child occasionally may be good, but giving them the chance to devour all the sweets and treats that they want could mean one big problem — childhood obesity.

Set the Limits

You do not know how to do it? Here are some tips that will help you keep track of your child's food and eating regimen and help him fight childhood obesity.

1.Happy Halloween!

As the only festival dedicated almost completely to overeating on "sugar laden treats," Halloween holds an extraordinary place in hell for most parents dealing with childhood obesity. This can understandably be a very tough time for your child to get through, but you can make it easier. Try focusing on the real spirit of the season and make a special haunted house for the kids, or let them have a "spooktacular" party with ghost stories, rubber spiders, and the old "spaghetti intestines and grape eyeballs" game. For younger kids, a costume party with pumpkin painting and other activities is always fun. The important thing is that you veer your kids away from any signs of sugary sweets.

2.Overnight Trips

The first solo sleepover can be nerve-wracking for both you and the host parents. Kids old enough for slumber parties and overnight trips are typically at least starting to manage some of their own food and diet regimen, which helps. Spend some time with the parents in advance of the event to give them a briefing on what your child might potentially need, and make yourself available via phone for any questions they might have. Provide them with healthy snacks that they can eat and give them nutritious foods to cook.

3.Calorie-Conscious Kiddos

It is important to teach your child about the kinds of foods that they are expected to eat. Splurge some time from your busy schedule, in teaching your child the comparative calorie counts of different foods. That will make your child make better food choices. It is better to teach them early how to read food labels to help boost their food awareness.

4.Snack on the Right Foods

Children are very vulnerable to snacks; hence, it would be difficult to remove them. The best way to prevent childhood obesity is to allow them to snack on the right foods. Give them some apples instead of a bar of chocolate. Keep in mind that eating is a habit. If your children's eating regimen has been accustomed to healthy eating from the very start, they will grow healthy and strong.

Indeed, fighting childhood obesity is not a problem. It is just in the manner parents teach their children about the right "stuffs" to eat.

Weight Loss Tips for Teens

Today's world puts a lot of extra pressure on teens to look thin. Popular TV shows aimed at teens all feature thin, pretty, young characters. Overbearing parents can put undue stress on their kids to lose weight… and even worse still, is that teenagers' peers can be incredibly judgmental of their weight. There's no easy solution to this problem. Weight loss is tough, and all the added anxiety that comes with being a teen only makes matters worse. Taking advantage of some of these pointers can help make the teenage experience less scary for overweight teens.

Healthy Eating Training for the Young

One of the most important tips, especially for young girls, is to make sure that you understand what a healthy person looks like. A lot of girls and young women on TV are, or at least appear, dangerously thin. The media may portray this as the ideal, but the truth is it's not a healthy lifestyle. Many young girls develop eating disorders trying to match the looks of women they see on TV, and this is a recipe for disaster. Young men can fall victim to eating disorders, too – it's not a problem exclusive to girls.

It's not uncommon for many teens to look in the mirror and see only ugliness and fat, when in reality they are a perfectly healthy young person. If you constantly feel severely depressed about your weight or your look, you should seek help from a psychologist. They can help you improve your own self-image and pursue weight loss goals in a healthy manner.

Understand What Your Body Has to Go Through

During your teen years, your body can undergo a number of changes that affect how you grow. For instance, you might hit a late growth spurt and gain a few inches in height, making your weight even out across your frame. Puberty is a complicated time – if you know that you're following a proper diet and exercise plan but aren't seeing results, you might just have to wait until you've fully grown into your body. Regardless of other factors, diet and exercise are always going to be an important factor in weight loss.

Keep this in mind as you go throughout your school day, and think of ways to improve your health.

- If your school cafeteria only serves greasy, unhealthy foods, talk to your parents about bringing a healthier lunch every day.

- Make sure to participate in gym class, and if you can, get involved in extra-curricular sports, too.

Teens Need Help

In almost every case, your family wants to be healthy too, and they will help you out as best they can. If one of your parents is the primary family cook, talk to them about healthier options for food. Furthermore, you can offer to help your parents with renovations or yard work for a little extra exercise.

These tips for weight loss for teens can make a huge difference for you.

Chapter 7- The Role Parents Play in Teen Weight Loss

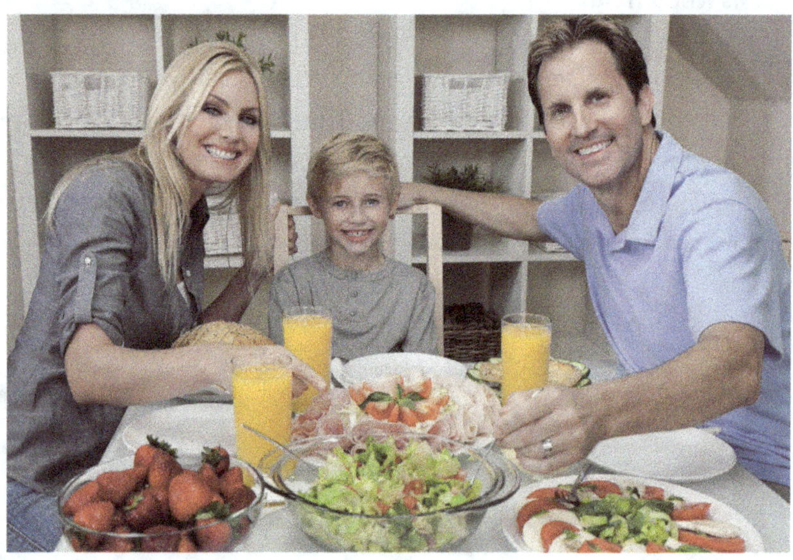

- Does your teen come home from school with tear-streaked cheeks, because of their weight?

- Do they rush to their bedroom because they don't want to talk about it?

- Are you crying with them because you know what they are going through?

It doesn't have to be that way for you or your teenager.

Recent studies have shown that teenage obesity has reached epidemic proportions. Most of these studies show that:

- Not only do body structure, DNA, diets of fast foods and overeating contribute to the weight problem,

- But the lack of physical activity, by today's adolescents, is a primary cause.

- Another fact revealed in these studies is that most young people still in their teens get less than 30 minutes of exercise in a 24 hour period.

Hey! Read on to learn about easy weight loss for teens!

Exercise

If you as a parent aren't exercising, you are contributing to your child's bad exercise habits and obesity. A good way to help yourself and your offspring, to get healthy, is to find an exercise program you can both do. As a matter of fact, it doesn't have to be a boring, repetitive type of exercise, but it can be one loaded with fun. However, there is one thing you should do before starting any exercise program.

Visit a Doctor

If both you and your teenager are overweight, it would pay for you to check with your doctor and your child's pediatrician. This physical checkup will rule out any underlying health problems which could be the cause of the weight gain. It will also determine if you're both healthy enough to engage in an exercise program to lose weight.

Weight Loss Doesn't Have to be Complicated

Believe it or not, you and your son or daughter, can start off with a walking program. To help make it bearable for the usual adolescent attitude, allow them to take along their I-pod or other music player. However, it's also a great time for you guys to have a good talk. You can actually ease into this over a period of days by talking about things that they are interested in. Don't use it as a time to preach at them, because if you do, not only will they block you out, you will kill whatever interest they have started to build in exercise.

Ride Bicycles and Swim

It is a great way to incorporate exercise into your life, while having a great time doing it. Family and friends can bike together, at parks, on bike trails, or almost any place that they choose. It is the perfect sport for anyone, no matter if they are 6 or 60. All they have to do is go at their own pace, because any speed is beneficial. As long as it gets the body moving and the blood pumping, it is providing a great health boost.

There is no excuse for someone not to ride a bike! Even if they've never learned how to ride a bike with two-wheels, there are adult-size tricycles which don't require balance to ride. All you do is hop on and start peddling.

The Different Sizes and Colors of Bikes

There are tiny tricycles for toddlers who are just learning what a bike is. Then there are regular two-wheel bikes with training wheels attached, for kids five and up who want to learn to ride. After they ride for a while with the training wheels on, and start to feel comfortable, they can then have an adult remove the training wheels so they can attempt to ride without them. It might possibly be scary for the child at first, and they will probably have a few falls and/or bruises, but they will soon discover that the fun and freedom bike riding was worth the effort.

After an older child has mastered bike riding, there are some other types of bikes that they can be tried out. Motorbikes, including kid-size motorcycles, are popular among youngsters. Some children feel that motorbikes are even more fun than traditional ones, but they're not getting the aerobic workout that they get from non-motor bikes. This is because there is no need to peddle; the motor does all the work.

Biking Accessories

A favorite among adults and children alike, are baskets. Baskets come in various shapes, colors and sizes, and can be attached on the front of the bike, near the handle bars, or on the back. Some other popular gadgets include: Lights, horns, pedometers and saddles, and many more.

Another fun exercise you both can participate in is swimming. Obviously not everyone has a private pool, but many health clubs, gyms, and other public places do.

You need to face the fact, as a parent, it is your overall responsibility to ensure your child's welfare and over health. By encouraging an exercise program now, while they are still young, will benefit them for the rest of their life. Easy weight loss for teens doesn't have to be hard, nor does it have to be boring. It just has to be done.

Losing Weight with Bowling

Bowling is a game sport that can free up your emotions. It can also be used to relieve stress and tension. It is perfect to those who are constantly busy with their lives and are frequently bombarded with pressure-filling jobs. But aside from these benefits, are you aware of other things that bowling can do for your body?

Of course, weight control with bowling is possible. After all, with this game sport, you get to move much of your body muscles. It makes you physically active, so you burn calories more as well. So, more than gaining higher physical vigor, you get some of your weight off, consequently giving you the fabulous body you so die for!

The Health Benefits of Bowling

The health benefits of weight control with bowling can be summarized into the following:

• Tone body muscles

Walking along the bowling lane, stretching your hand to attempt making a spare or strike, and releasing the weighty ball are enough to promote good muscle exercises. This is just like when you exercise by walking, but with bowling there is weight involved; thus, you get more of the exercise. The stretching or flexing of your hand is also a good way for your joints, ligaments, tendons, and muscles to get good exercise. In addition, it also promotes good blood circulation. So, overall, bowling is a fun way of exercising and losing weight in the process.

• Burn fats

As you continue to move with those walking, flexing, stretching, and swinging; you are already causing some accumulated calories or fats to get burned. So, continuous involvement in this sport can be a routine of weight loss.

• Build Friendships

You get to bond with your friends, family, or relatives with continuous engagement with bowling trips. You create good social relationships, which are psychologically known to promote better heart performance. A better heart performance is great match with weight loss or control.

Lose the Weight but Keep the Fun

A personal experience, but apply this to your child's life! Now, I am not sure about you, but many people find it so hard to diet and to lose weight. This is the way it was for my husband. The weight loss programs and diets that he had tried were, to him, just so boring. They were also very hard for him to implement, as they were asking him to give up foods that he knew that he would not be able to stay away from. What we need is a weight loss program that is actually fun to put into action!

My husband's weight problems began when his parents decided to turn vegetarian. He was eleven years of age at the time and basically decided to give it a go as well. His mom cooked the meals, you see, so I guess he didn't have much choice. This was many years ago and at that point there were not many different options of food for people who were vegetarians.

He was not at all impressed with the food he was given and missed eating meat in a big way. He would normally be hungry after meals and would then start to eat snack type foods. He only gradually put on more weight, and people did not really comment for a couple of years.

Obesity is a Vicious Cycle

As soon as people did notice, it was like a vicious circle. They would taunt my husband at school. He would come home all depressed and would then "comfort eat," to make himself feel better.

A few years ago he went about looking for ways to help him to lose weight. He tried many diets but without success. I have to say it was not that anything was wrong with the actual diets he was trying; it was that any given particular diet did not suit him. He is the type of person who needs to enjoy something to keep his interest in it. This is why he found school a struggle. Well, that is his excuse anyway, I gently tease him.

On a Saturday night a few years ago, my husband went out for a night out with a good friend of his (Dave). They were having a good chat during which he told Dave about his mission to lose weight. He explained about how, as yet, he had not found a suitable weight loss program.

Compete

Dave suggested that my husband should take up a sport, something competitive that he could get his teeth into. He thought about what Dave had said and agreed that this could be the way to go. He asked Dave if he would like a game of tennis three or four times a week. Dave stated that this might be a bit much, as he played six-a-side football twice a week.

Dave did not want to let my husband down, however, and then asked if my husband would like to join his six-a-side team. "I will give it a go," my husband replied. My husband came home a bit giddy and also rather pleased with himself. He now had a weight loss plan that he was sure would work. There will be no quick fix;

this amount of exercise, over a sustained period of time, would have a positive effect on his weight, his fitness, and his health.

It did take quite a while, as my husband had predicted, to reach a weight that he was happy with. This was not a problem however, as he was having fun on the way.

He continues to play not only tennis and football, but many sports. This is no longer to lose weight but because he enjoys it tremendously. And so will your teen!

Chapter 8- Correcting Mindsets, Correcting Weight Issues

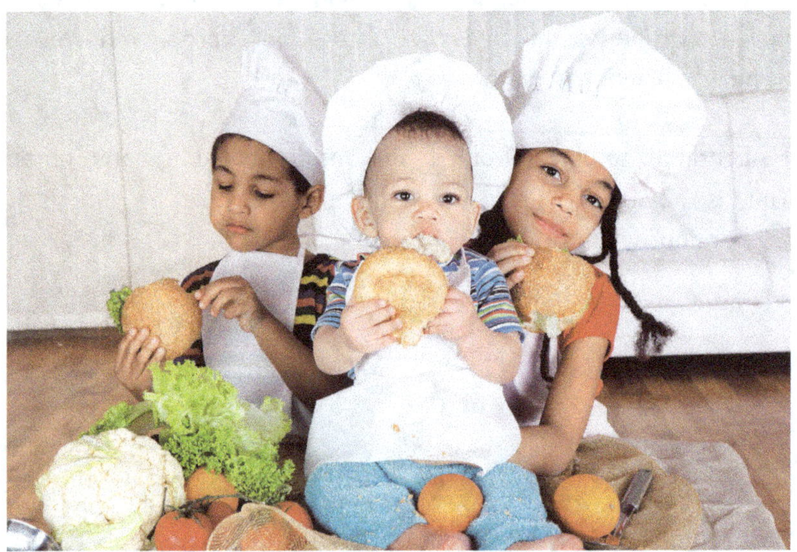

Worried about your daughter's eating habits? Overall, teenage girls are more likely to diet and be concerned about their weight than their male peers, regardless of age and whether the girls were actually overweight.

Start Early

Living a healthy life is one of the major keys to a joyful life, and living a healthy lifestyle must start in the early years. In many instances, good parenting will, many times, start children off on the correct foot. Often, however, it will call for more effort. If you have a teen girl who suffers from being overweight, you may need to do "above and beyond" to help them. Weight loss for teenage girls oftentimes is a complex hurdle to jump alone.

Nancy Green
The "I'm Involved" Mindset

They require compassionate parents who can maintain fit home environments — and who provide excellent role models. When parents do well at losing weight, their kids are more prone to succeeding, as well. If you are inclined toward dramatic weight fluctuations and widely varying diets, your daughter will attempt to follow your lead. As you no doubt agree, a growing young person will not benefit emotionally, physically, or nutritionally from this type of weight management.

The mixture of obesity as an emerging epidemic among young people, and the stress on being thin-to-emaciated for teenage girls makes weight loss a most important issue.

To help a teen girl to lose weight, remember these years can be highly charged and emotional, particularly if a girl feels different from the others. Talk to a teen about eating healthier foods instead of simply giving up eating to lose weight. The only way a teenage girl should achieve a healthy weight is by eating in a well-balanced, moderate and healthful manner.

Does an Extremely Low Calorie Diet Help?

Ironically, extreme low calorie dieting among teenagers typically leads to an increase in weight, instead of weight loss. After a brief episode of swift initial loss in weight, the body and metabolism begin to slow down, with the purpose of conserving calories. This is a natural body defense system, intended to rise above the effects of a food deficiency. This path will only harm, and never help your daughter. New research indicates that eating at least five meals together as a family, per week, significantly decreases the odds of teenage girls engaging in acute diet behaviors, such as fasting or anorexic/bulimic actions such as vomiting.

Think about the culture that today's teenage girls are wrapped up in – a way of life that deifies extremely thin models and actresses. Your daughter only sees the "PhotoShop'ed" images for the media, and not the realities or the hardships that even these women suffer. Your teenage girl probably is comparing herself to those models and actresses… and most certainly has unrealistic beliefs about how her own body should appear.

For beginners, your daughter should not panic. There are safe ways of fighting toward weight loss, and this can only begin to happen with the assistance of a professional. Perhaps some counseling is in order… but a better place to start may be with simple measures of appealing to her good sense of nutrition and feeling good!

Help Your Child Plan Her Own Success

Consider taking your teenage girl to a nutritionist, who will help in developing a levelheaded weight-loss plan.

Let your daughter be a part of her own plan! The nutritionist is an unbiased third party, and can offer suggestions to your girl about how she might improve her food habits, without imposing any guilt on her.

Chapter 9- Helping Your Overweight Teenage Boys

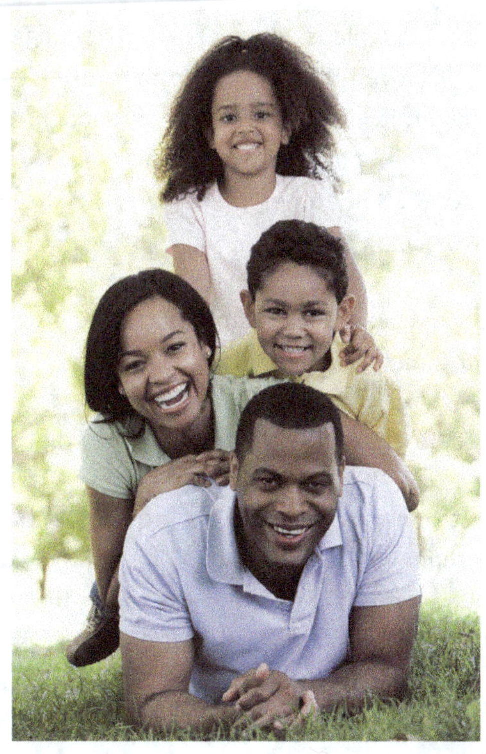

If you have been looking for diet plans for overweight teenage boys, then you are in luck. Many teenage boys are overweight, even some of the more active ones. From football players to baseball players, overweight teenage boys can be found doing all sorts of different things. It does not matter what race they are or what types of activities they do or what all they eat for supper. Overweight teenage boys can be found from all walks of life.

Many people have a stereotypical idea that all overweight teenage boys indulge in video games for hours upon end, and simply do not get the proper exercise that is required in order to help maintain a healthy body weight. Unfortunately, this is not always the case. Even in teenage boys that participate in active sports, some will find themselves still being overweight. Whether they play tennis, golf, baseball, or chess, these overweight teenage boys are found in each and every niche.

Finding the right diet plans for overweight teenage boys can be extremely difficult. Even if you find the right exercise plan for the particular teenager, it might simply not be enough. One might try to resort to other methods, such as diet pills, but this is not always the best way to go. Sometimes the answer can be much simpler than to resort to buying diet pills.

Sometimes, the answer is as simple as taking a combination of actions in order to help that teenager lose weight.

1. Ensure that the teenager is on a good, healthy diet.

Remember that teenagers are always growing, and so they need more energy than you might think. This can make it hard to determine just how much is too much, but with time and patience, and a little luck, you can usually determine what is just right for your specific teenager. Not only should you pay attention to how much is in the diet, but you must also pay attention to what is in the diet.

2. Vitamins and dietary supplements may be needed.

Vitamin and other dietary supplements can help to ensure that your teenager is getting all of the vitamins and nutrients he needs, though you cannot depend entirely on them.

3. Get him on an exercise plan

After having determined the right diet for your teenager, try to get him on an exercise plan that helps to ensure that he is active. If he is already involved in active sports, then this, combined with his new healthy diet, should help to ensure that your teenager begins to lose weight.

It can be truly amazing how much of a difference dieting and exercise when combined can make in a teenage boy's life, or in the lives of others. He will have more energy and be more confident in himself and his abilities. Diet plans for overweight teenage boys can be the perfect way to motivate your teenager and help him feel good about himself.

CHAPTER 10- FUN DIET RECIPES FOR TEENS AND MOMS

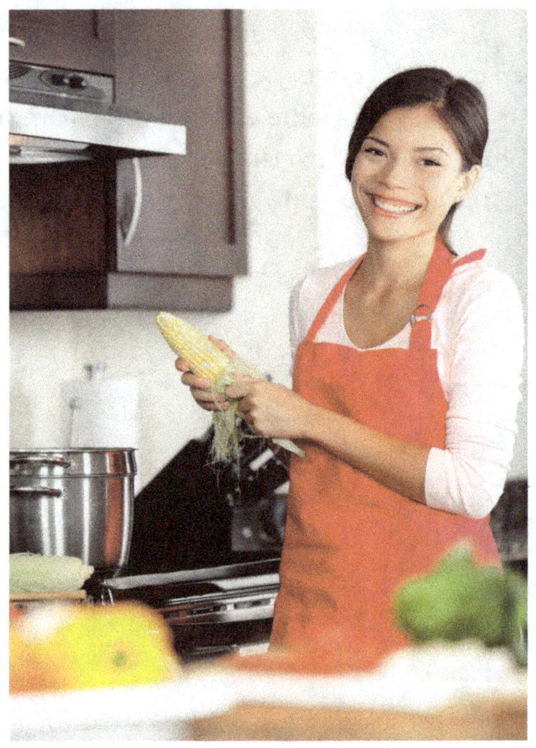

Wow. It just seems like all of us are dieting these days! This will help YOU, if you are the one dieting. But, hiding in the corners is also the base for making sure that your kids are eating well and off to a good start in life, as well! If you are a mom on a diet, you will probably relate to a very frequent situation.

Many moms with children are able to keep to a healthy eating plan through most circumstances except two. It all starts to go astray when the kids come home from school, or when they are preparing school lunches. It's no surprise really. Kids love snacks we buy from the supermarket, and parents love them because they are quick and easy to throw into the lunchbox or for kids to grab from the shelves in the pantry. Small bags of chips, tasty bite size crackers, sodas, and the like. No problem. Except when it comes to moms weight loss program. These products are high in fat, high in energy, and high in refined sugars. And after one, two, or three nibbles, it is possible to rack up an unwanted 500 calories. This single act will probably stall your weight loss or even worse!

To stop your kids from sabotaging your weight loss efforts, here are 20 snack ideas for kids that will do far less damage to your weight loss program if mom nibbles (just a little).

1. Chop up ½ tinned pears or other fruit in natural juice and set in 200mls of low calorie jelly. Make up into individual disposable plastic containers with lids.

2. Cut up crisp vegetable sticks with dipping sauce – ranch, peanut (satay), sweet chili or tomato.

3. Cut celery sticks 6-8 cm, fill with cottage cheese and top with sultanas or chopped nuts.

4. Combine a mixture of low fat hard cheese cubes, nuts and dried fruits in plastic wrap or a lunch bag.

5. Roll up thin slices of carrot and celery with grated cheese in a slice of cold meat. Secure with toothpick. Slice the carrot and celery with a vegetable peeler for really thin slices.

6. Cut oranges into quarters and freeze on trays. Put into plastic bags for a fruity ice block.

7. Meatball surprise. Next time you are making meatloaf, double the quantity and make a batch of meatballs. These are great in lunchboxes cold. Add a slice of pineapple with a toothpick to each meatball. Add dipping tomato sauce if required.

8. Mini quiches….make a batch of crust-less quiche and cook in muffin tray. Each 'muffin' will be a wonderful healthy snack for kids.

9. Chilled fruit surprise – slice a combination of strawberries, bananas, kiwi fruit, watermelon, grapes or in season fruit. Place in small resealable plastic container. Top with apple juice; do not overfill. Seal then freeze. When packed in lunchbox, will keep sandwiches cool and prove a refreshing treat on a hot day.

10. Rice cakes spread with mashed avocado, mashed banana and cinnamon, or try mashed avocado, sliced tomato and sprouts.

11. Chopped hard-boiled egg served with low fat mayo, salt, pepper on crisp bread.

12. Leaf wrappers: wrap a cheese finger, celery stick and carrot stick in a lettuce leaf. Wrap in foil and place in lunchbox. Contents will be kept moist.

13. Yoghurt tub.

14. Baby Bell Cheese and low fat cracker.

15. Creamy dates: slice dates lengthways, remove stone. Fill with Philadelphia cream cheese (low fat).

16. Quick sausage rolls: wrap a skinned (good quality) sausage in several sheets of filo pastry. Brush pastry with beat egg to glaze. Cut into desired lengths. Bake in moderately hot oven for 15-20 minutes. Rolls can be frozen.

17. Same as above but use fresh chicken breast strips and cut to 2" – use tomato or favorite dipping sauce

18. After school hot snack attack: Spread a round of pita bread with tomato paste and herbs. Top with tomato, ham, mortadella (large Italian sausage), add onion, sliced mushrooms or pineapple. Sprinkle grated low fat hard cheese over pita bread. Grill to make a tasty pizza. If no pita bread is available, substitute crisp bread.

19. Fruity kebabs: place bite size pieces of fruit in season on kebab skewers.

20. Pop top sandwich tuna tin, crisp bread, sachet of mayonnaise. Kids can put their snack together at school so that it doesn't go soggy.

Remember, fresh is best, both for yourself and your children. By substituting these ideas for some of the prepackaged snack food and cookies your kids eat, you will be doing both them and yourself a favor.

About the Author

Nancy Green is a mother of two and a nutritionist. She specializes in childhood obesity.

Armed with knowledge from first-hand experiences, Nancy knows what it's like living with too much weight. She was obese herself growing up in Bronx, New York. She has had many hospital trips because of her deteriorating health caused by obesity. When she finally managed to control her weight, she reported said feeling relieved.

Today, Nancy is an active advocate of health and wellness.